I0767751

Pancreatic/Prostate Cancer

How you get rid of pancreatic or prostate cancer and reclaim your healthy lifestyle.

By

Lucille R. Breed

Disclaimer

In case you purchase this book without a cover or purchase a PDF, JPG, or spat copy of it, it is splendidly taken property or a phony. Taking into account everything, neither the makers, the merchant, nor any of their laborers or experts have gotten any piece of the copy. Besides, mutilating is a known street to financial assistance for laborers with horrible approaches to acting and mental aggressor parties. We request that you not buy any such copies and report any event of someone offering such copies to Plata Appropriating LLC.

This dispersing is needed to give talented and strong information concerning the subject covered. Anyway, is sold with the appreciation that the maker and vendor have not taken part in conveying true blue, cash-related, or other master direction. Rules and practices at times change starting with one state and then onto the accompanying and country to country, and assuming authentic or other expert assistance is required, the relationship of a specialist should be searched for.

The essayist and merchant unequivocally disavow any liability that is accomplished by the utilization or utilization of the things in this book.

Copyright © 2024 by Lucille R. Breed. All rights reserved.

Safeguarded by safeguarded development rules. Also, as permitted under the U.S. Copyright Show of 1976, no piece of this transport may be copied, dispersed, sent in any arrangement or utilizing all means, or set aside in an instructive combination or recuperation system without the previous assent of the wholesaler.
Dispersed by **Lucille R. Breed.**

Introduction

At any point do you accept that individuals passed because they have Disease? All that you catch wind of bosom disease is false.

Certain individuals do accept that malignant growth spells almost certain doom for the street, yet it's not the very thing you think.

Malignant growth can be a perilous infection yet it doesn't mean it will kill you.

Hi everybody! I go by **Lucille R. Breed,** I'm an individual of 62 years of age from Dallas.

I was a specialist in a clinic in Forney when I was 31 years of age, I had pancreatic disease and I was unable to treat it at my clinic, and this made me think I planned to pass on, I went through a few medical procedures and there was no solution for malignant growth, I began living in dread and agony feel that is the stopping point for me. On one occasion I met a lady in Euless who was a pancreatic malignant growth trained professional, following fourteen days of therapy I got from her, I recuperated from the disease and I became solid and sound till this exact second I'm very well solid.

After I recuperated from malignant growth, I chose to begin working with her, and I worked with her for just about 24 years.

Dear peruser! The items in this book are stringently to tell you how to forestall pancreatic disease and how to be aware assuming you are creating malignant growth side effects at a beginning phase.

The items in this book are precisely the things I have encountered, learned, and shown individuals who created pancreatic disease around me and it has turned out great for them. I chose to compose this book in other to contact more individuals out there and to save additional individuals from malignant growth sickness. Individuals have been giving declarations from my instructing and you can likewise be a piece of them by getting yourself a duplicate of this book. Remain Favored.

Table of contacts

Chapter One

Pancreatic Disease

What is pancreatic disease?

The pancreas assumes a fundamental part in assimilation by delivering catalysts that the body needs to process fats, starches, and proteins.

The pancreas additionally delivers two significant chemicals: glucagon and insulin. These chemicals are liable for controlling glucose (sugar) digestion. Insulin assists cells with utilizing glucose to make energy, and glucagon helps raise glucose levels when they are excessively low.

There are two fundamental sorts of pancreatic disease, in light of the sort of cell they start in:

Pancreatic adenocarcinoma. This is the most well-known kind of pancreatic disease. It begins in exocrine cells, which produce compounds that guide processing.

Pancreatic neuroendocrine cancers. This more extraordinary sort of pancreatic disease begins in the endocrine cells, which discharge chemicals that influence everything from the state of mind to digestion.

Pancreatic disease side effects

Pancreatic disease frequently doesn't cause side effects until it arrives at cutting-edge stages. Thus, there ordinarily aren't any early indications of pancreatic disease.

Indeed, even at further developed stages, probably the most widely recognized pancreatic disease side effects can be unobtrusive.

As it advances, pancreatic disease can cause the accompanying side effects:

loss of hunger

accidental weight reduction

stomach torment, which could transmit to your back

lower back torment

blood clusters (frequently in the leg, which can cause redness, agony, and enlarging)

jaundice (yellowing skin and eyes)

wretchedness

light-hued or oily stools

dim or brown pee

irritated skin

queasiness

retching

Pancreatic malignant growth can likewise influence your glucose. At times, this could prompt diabetes (or the deterioration of prior diabetes).

Remember that the above side effects can be brought about by a scope of less serious well-being concerns.

Pancreatic malignant growth causes

The reason for pancreatic malignant growth is obscure.

Pancreatic disease happens when strange cells start to develop inside the pancreas and structure grows, however, it's indistinct why this works out.

Ordinarily, sound cells develop and bite the dust in moderate numbers. On account of malignant growth, there's an expansion in the creation of unusual cells. These cells ultimately take over solid cells.

While the basic reason for pancreatic malignant growth is obscure, certain variables might build your gamble of creating it.

These include:
Tobacco use. Smoking cigarettes might represent 20 to 35 percent confided in Source of pancreatic malignant growth cases.

Weighty liquor utilization. Having at least three cocktails daily might build your gamble. Drinking liquor can likewise add to pancreatitis, another gambling factor.

Constant and inherited pancreatitis. This alludes to the aggravation of the pancreas. Constant pancreatitis frequently results from weighty drinking over an extensive period. Pancreatitis can likewise be genetic.

Weight. Having overweight or corpulence, especially in early adulthood, may expand your gamble.

Diet. Eating an eating routine high in red and handled meats, seared food varieties, sugar, or cholesterol might expand your gamble, however, specialists are as yet sorting out the specific connection between dietary variables and pancreatic disease risk.

Sex. Men are somewhat more certain to foster pancreatic disease than ladies.
Work environment openness. Working with specific synthetic compounds, especially those utilized in metalworking, and pesticides might be a calculation of up to 12 percent of pancreatic malignant growth cases.

Age. Individuals between the ages of 65 and 74 are bound to be determined to have pancreatic malignant growth.

Diabetes. You might have a higher gamble of creating pancreatic disease if you have type 1 or type 2 diabetes.

Race. In the US, paces of pancreatic disease are most elevated among Individuals of color. Research from 2018 recommends this is because of a blend of way of life, financial, and hereditary variables, however, specialists note a requirement for more examination concerning the fundamental reasons for racial differences in paces of pancreatic malignant growth.

Family ancestry. Up to 10 percent of individuals with pancreatic malignant growth have a family background of the condition.

Contaminations. Having a past filled with H. pylori contamination in your gastrointestinal system might build your gamble, however, the specific connection to pancreatic disease isn't clear. Having hepatitis B may likewise expand your gamble by up to 24 percent.

Certain hereditary varieties and changes can cause conditions that may likewise build your gamble of pancreatic disease.

A portion of these circumstances include:

Peutz-Jeghers condition

Lynch condition

familial abnormal various mole melanoma disorder

acquired pancreatitis

inherited bosom and ovarian malignant growth disorder

Pancreatic disease determination

Early conclusion altogether builds the possibilities of recuperation. That is the reason it's ideal to consider a medical care proficient to be soon as could be expected assuming that you notice any surprising side effects, particularly if you have any gamble factors for pancreatic disease.

To conclude, your consideration group will survey your side effects and clinical history. They might arrange at least one test to check for pancreatic disease, for example,

CT or X-ray outputs to get a total and definite picture of your pancreas

an endoscopic ultrasound, where a flimsy, adaptable cylinder with a camera joined is embedded down into the stomach to get pictures of the pancreas

biopsy, or tissue test, of the pancreas

blood tests to distinguish assuming growth marker CA 19-9 is available, which can show pancreatic disease

Pancreatic malignant growth stages

At the point when pancreatic disease is found, specialists will probably play out extra tests to decide if the malignant growth has spread. These could incorporate imaging tests, like a PET sweep, or blood tests.

They'll utilize the consequences of these tests to lay out the phase of the malignant growth. Arranging makes sense of how exceptional the disease is, which will assist with deciding the best treatment choice.

The phases of pancreatic malignant growth are:

Stage 0. There are strange cells in the pancreas that could become dangerous. This stage is some of the time called precancer.

Stage 1. The growth is just in the pancreas.

Stage 2. The cancer has spread to local stomach tissues or lymph hubs.

Stage 3. The growth has spread to significant veins and lymph hubs.

Stage 4. The cancer has spread to different organs, similar to the liver. This is likewise called metastatic malignant growth.

Here is a more critical glance at the various phases of pancreatic disease.

Pancreatic malignant growth stage 4

Stage 4 pancreatic malignant growth has spread past the first site to far-off locales, such as different organs, the mind, or bones.

Pancreatic malignant growth is frequently analyzed at this late stage since it seldom causes side effects until it has spread to different destinations.

Side effects you could insight at this stage include:

torment in the upper midsection

torment toward the back

weakness

jaundice (yellowing of the skin)

a deficiency of craving

weight reduction

melancholy

Stage 4 pancreatic malignant growth can't be restored, however therapies can alleviate side effects and keep difficulties from the disease.

Pancreatic malignant growth stage 3

Stage 3 pancreatic malignant growth is a cancer in the pancreas and conceivably close by destinations, like lymph hubs or veins.

Side effects of stage 3 pancreatic malignant growth might include:

torment toward the back

agony or delicacy in the upper midsection

a deficiency of hunger

weight reduction

weariness

despondency

Stage 3 pancreatic disease is challenging to fix, however therapies can assist with forestalling the spread of the malignant growth and simplicity side effects.

These medicines might include: medical procedures to eliminate a part of the pancreas
anticancer medications
radiation treatment
Most of the individuals with this phase of malignant growth will have a repeat. That is reasonable because of the way that micrometastases, or little areas of imperceptible disease development, have spread past the pancreas at the hour of identification and aren't taken out during a medical procedure.

Pancreatic malignant growth stage 2

Stage 2 pancreatic malignant growth is a disease that remaining parts of the pancreas however may have spread to a couple of neighboring lymph hubs or veins.

This stage is partitioned into two subcategories, contingent upon where the disease is and the size of the growth:

Stage 2A. The growth is bigger than 4 centimeters (cm) yet hasn't spread to any lymph hubs or nearby tissue.

Stage 2B. The cancer has spread to local lymph hubs, however not to more than three of them.

Side effects of stage 2 pancreatic malignant growth will generally be extremely inconspicuous and may include:

jaundice

changes in pee tone

agony or delicacy in the upper mid-region

weight reduction

loss of hunger

weariness

Treatment might include:

medical procedure

radiation

chemotherapy

designated drug treatments

Your PCP might utilize a blend of these ways to deal with assistance contract the growth and forestall potential metastases.

Pancreatic disease stage 1

Stage 1 pancreatic disease includes a cancer that is just in the pancreas. This stage is separated into two subcategories, contingent upon the size of the cancer:

Stage 1A. The cancer estimates 2 cm or less.

Stage 1B. The growth estimates multiple cm however under 4 cm.

Stage 1 pancreatic disease regularly causes no perceptible side effects.

Whenever distinguished at this stage, pancreatic disease might be reparable with medical procedures.

Pancreatic malignant growth stage 0

This is the earliest phase of pancreatic malignant growth, however it may not be guaranteed to include disease. It simply implies that strange cells have been distinguished, and they might become dangerous later on. This stage includes no side effects.

Chapter Two

Pancreatic disease treatment

Treating pancreatic disease includes two principal objectives: to kill harmful cells and keep the malignant growth from spreading. The most fitting therapy choice will rely upon the phase of the disease.

The principal treatment choices include:
Medical procedure. Careful therapy of pancreatic malignant growth includes eliminating segments of the pancreas (more on this beneath). While this can dispose of the first growth, it won't eliminate disease that is spread to different regions. Therefore, medical procedure ordinarily isn't suggested for cutting-edge stage pancreatic disease.
Radiation treatment. X-beams and other high-energy radiates are utilized to kill malignant growth cells.

Chemotherapy. Anticancer medications are utilized to kill disease cells and assist with forestalling their future development.

Designated treatment. Prescriptions and antibodies are utilized to separately target disease cells without hurting different cells, which can occur with chemotherapy and radiation treatment.

Immunotherapy. Different strategies are utilized to set off your safe framework to focus on the disease.

At times, a specialist could suggest consolidating numerous treatment choices. For instance, chemotherapy may be finished before a medical procedure.

For cutting-edge stage pancreatic malignant growth, treatment choices could zero in more on relief from discomfort and keeping side effects as sensible as could be expected.

Pancreatic malignant growth medical procedure

Growths restricted to the "head and neck" of the pancreas can be eliminated with a strategy called the Whipple method (pancreaticoduodenectomy).

In this methodology, the initial segment, or the "head" of the pancreas, and around 20% of the "body," or the subsequent part, is eliminated. The base portion of the bile channel and the initial segment of the digestive system is likewise taken out.

In a changed form of this medical procedure, a piece of the stomach is likewise taken out.

Pancreatic disease future and endurance rate

An endurance rate is a level of the number of individuals with the very type and phase of a disease that is as yet alive after a particular measure of time. This number doesn't show how long individuals might live. All things considered, it helps check how fruitful therapy for malignant growth may be.

Numerous endurance rates are given as a 5-year rate, which alludes to the level of individuals alive 5 years in the wake of being analyzed or beginning treatment.

It's essential to remember that endurance rates aren't conclusive and can shift significantly from one individual to another depending upon age, generally speaking, well-being, and how the malignant growth advances. Subsequently, they likewise can't decide a singular's future.

Endurance rates for pancreatic malignant growth are ordinarily accommodated in confined, territorial, and far-off stages:
Confined. The disease hasn't spread from the pancreas, which relates to stages 0, 1, or 2A.

Territorial. Malignant growth has spread to local tissues or lymph hubs, which relates to stages 2B and 3.

Far off. Disease has spread to far-off locales, similar to the lungs or bones, which relates to stage 4.

Here is a glance at the 1-, 5-, and 10-year relative endurance rates from finding for each stage.

Stage
1-year endurance rate
5-year endurance rate

10-year endurance rate

Limited
55%
35.4%
29.8%
Provincial
50.6%
12.3%
8.1%
Far off
17.4%
2.8%
1.6%

Assuming that you or a friend or family member was as of late determined to have pancreatic disease, it's justifiable to promptly ponder the future, yet this relies upon a scope of elements that differ extraordinarily from one individual to another. Your medical services group can give the most dependable gauge given these elements.

Pancreatic malignant growth guess

Endurance rates must depend on individuals who have first treated something like a long time back.

Somebody being analyzed today might have a superior endurance rate thanks to progress in disease medicines.

All things considered, pancreatic malignant growth is as yet viewed as challenging to treat, to a great extent since it frequently isn't found until it's spread to different pieces of the body.

Racial contrasts in anticipation: Dark Americans aren't simply bound to foster pancreatic malignant growth more than white Americans. They're additionally more likely to bite the dust from the condition.

Research from 2019 recommends a critical piece of this dissimilarity is driven by imbalances in treatment. Specialists likewise highlight long-haul racial separation, especially as isolation, as a driving variable.

Pancreatic malignant growth avoidance

It's as yet not satisfactory what causes pancreatic malignant growth, so there's no dependable method for forestalling it.

While specific things could expand your gamble of creating pancreatic disease, a portion of these — like your family ancestry and age — can't be changed.

Be that as it may, a couple of way of life changes might assist with diminishing your gamble:

Stop smoking. Assuming that you presently smoke, investigate various ways to deal with assistance you quit.

Limit liquor. Weighty drinking might expand your gamble of constant pancreatitis and, perhaps, pancreatic malignant growth.

Keep a moderate weight. A scope of variables can add to overweight and corpulence, some of which you have zero control over. If you are overweight or hefty, consider consulting with a medical services professional about procedures for keeping a moderate weight.

Integrate entire food sources. Certain food sources, including red meat, handled meat, sugar, and seared food varieties, may expand your gamble of pancreatic malignant growth. You don't have to remove these from your eating regimen, yet intend to offset them with new or frozen leafy foods, entire grains, and lean proteins.

Chapter Three

Prostate Cancer

What's prostate cancer?

Prostate malignant growth is the most regularly analyzed disease in guys around the world. In the US, the American Malignant Growth Society (ACS) appraises that 268,490 men will be recently determined to have this condition in 2022.

The prostate is a little organ tracked down in a man's lower midsection, situated under the bladder and encompassing the urethra. The chemical testosterone directs the prostate. Moreover, the prostate organ produces the original liquid, otherwise called semen.

Semen is the substance containing sperm that leaves the urethra during discharge.

At the point when a strange, harmful development of cells — which is known as a growth — structures in the prostate, it's called prostate disease. This disease can spread to different regions of the body. In these

cases, because the malignant growth is made of cells from the prostate, it's called prostate disease.

Sorts of prostate disease

Practically all instances of prostate disease are a sort of malignant growth called adenocarcinoma that fills in the tissue of an organ, like the prostate organ. In any case, other uncommon sorts of disease can likewise start in the prostate, including:

little cell carcinoma, like a cellular breakdown in the lungs

neuroendocrine growths, like pancreatic disease

momentary cell carcinomas, like kidney malignant growth

sarcomas, like bone cell disease

Prostate disease is additionally classified by how quickly it develops. It has two kinds of development:

forceful, or quickly developing

nonaggressive, or slow-developing

With nonaggressive prostate disease, the cancer develops gradually. In any case, with forceful disease, the growth can congest and spread to other body regions, like the bones, and turn into a metastatic malignant growth.

Prostate disease causes and hazard factors

There's no known reason for prostate disease, however, risk factors, for example, family ancestry or age might improve your probability of fostering the harm.

Who's in danger?

While prostate malignant growth could happen in any man, certain variables raise your gamble for the illness. These gamble factors include:

more established age, 50 years old or more established

family background of prostate disease

certain nationalities or races — for example, African American guys are at a more serious gamble of having prostate malignant growthbcorpulence hereditary changes

A few investigations consider other gambling factors like eating routine and compound openness that might build your finding possibilities. Notwithstanding, the ACS says those impacts are as

yet hazy. Prostate disease is likewise uncommon in men younger than 40.

Prostate disease side effects

A few types of prostate disease are nonaggressive, so you might not have any side effects. Nonetheless, the high-level prostate disease frequently causes side effects.

If you have any of the accompanying signs or side effects, make it a point to your primary care physician. Moreover, different circumstances can cause a few side effects of prostate malignant growth, like harmless prostatic hyperplasia (BPH), so you'll have to check with your PCP to get a legitimate finding.

Side effects of prostate malignant growth can incorporate urinary issues, sexual issues, and torment and deadness.

Urinary issues

Urinary issues are normal because the prostate is situated underneath the bladder and encompasses the urethra. In light of this area, on the off chance that cancer develops on the prostate, it could push on the bladder or urethra and create issues.

Urinary issues can include:

regular need to pee

a stream that is slower or more fragile than typical

draining while at the same time peeing

Sexual issues

Erectile brokenness might be a side effect of prostate disease. Additionally called feebleness, this condition makes you incapable to get and keep an erection.

Blood in the semen after discharge can likewise be a side effect of prostate malignant growth.

Torment and deadness

You might encounter shortcomings or deadness in the legs and feet. You may likewise fail to keep a grip on your bladder and gut on the off chance that the disease has spread, causing strain on your spinal line.

Early location of prostate malignant growth

One of the most incredible ways of identifying malignant growth before any side effects seem is to go through a screening test. The previous you find the disease, the more straightforward it could be to treat.

Prostate-explicit antigen (public service announcement)

Public service announcement is a blood test that affects the quantity of prostate proteins in your blood. Assuming the level is high, it might show prostate malignant growth.

The public service announcement test is a helpful instrument for your PCP to consider whether your public service announcement levels might demonstrate prostate malignant growth. Since early discovery is critical for treating disease, this is a significant advantage. The test is moderately straightforward and broadly accessible for individuals with a prostate that needs to be screened. Notwithstanding, there are upsides and downsides to screening. For instance, a recent report found that public service announcements might build your possibilities of early identification, however, it doesn't diminish your possibilities of biting the dust from prostate malignant growth. The test has a few related concerns and it is vital to examine with your primary care physician what the dangers of public service announcement screening would mean for you.

Different worries to consider about public service announcements include:

exactness level

overdiagnosis and overtreatment propensities

indistinct in general advantage

Different variables can expand your public service announcement level, for example,

expanded prostate

more established age

discharge

prostate contamination or irritation

explicit drugs

Advanced rectal test (DRE)

At the point when you go through a DRE, the specialist puts their greased-up, gloved finger into your rectum to feel any knocks, unbending, or broadened region of the prostate.

Since prostate malignant growth frequently begins at the rear of the organ, it very well might be identified utilizing this strategy. Albeit not generally so viable as a public service announcement test, it is more powerful among men who have a typical public service announcement level yet at the same time have prostate malignant growth.

Prostate imaging

Utilizing progressed imaging, for example, X-ray or ultrasound, you can distinguish prostate disease. In a 2018 exploration article, specialists showed that you

can now get it prior — and better distinguish its stage — with further developed innovations.

Prostate biopsy

At times, your PCP might suggest a prostate biopsy on the off chance that they suspect disease from a test or find that you have a raised public service announcement level.

During the biopsy, the specialist takes a little example of your prostate tissue to dissect the phones. If they find the cells are malignant, it can likewise assist them with deciding how rapidly they might spread and develop. To do this, they decide your Gleason score.

The Gleason score is a viable apparatus to foresee your viewpoint, yet it isn't outright. There are numerous different variables included while anticipating the spread and course of the sickness, with specialists shifting by the way they utilize the scoring framework.

Undoubtedly, the most ideal way to decide your viewpoint relies upon different indicators notwithstanding your Gleason scores, similar to your actual test and growth imaging

Prostate malignant growth screening by age

The ACS has evaluated proposals for men as they age.

To begin with, they prescribe that specialists converse with men about the upsides and downsides of screening prostate malignant growth during a yearly test. These discussions ought to happen for the following ages:

Age 40: For men at extremely high gamble, like those with more than one first-degree relative — a dad, sibling, or child — who had prostate malignant growth at an age more youthful than 65.

Age 45: For men at high gamble, for example, African American men and men with a first-degree relative analyzed at an age more youthful than 65.

Age 50: For men at normal gamble of prostate disease, and who are supposed to inhabit at least 10 additional years.

Before you choose to go through screening, consider all the data accessible, including vulnerabilities, dangers, and advantages of prostate malignant growth screening. Then, you and your PCP can conclude which test is best for you, if any.

Prostate disease stages

Your PCP can examine how far the disease has spread by utilizing an organizing framework.

The American Joint Advisory Group on Malignant Growth (AJCC) TMN arranging framework stages prostate disease. In the same way as other different kinds of malignant growth, the framework stages it by:

the size or degree of the growth

lymph hub contribution

whether malignant growth has spread (metastasized) to different destinations or organs

Public service announcement level at the hour of analysis

Gleason score

Prostate malignant growth stages range from 1 to 4. Nonetheless, the illness is most developed in stage 4.

Prostate disease treatment

Your PCP will foster a suitable therapy plan for your malignant growth in light of your age, well-being status, and the phase of your disease.

Nonaggressive

If the disease is nonaggressive, your primary care physician might suggest vigilant pausing, likewise

called dynamic reconnaissance. This implies you'll postpone therapy yet have normal exams with your primary care physician to screen for malignant growth.

Assuming that your PCP decides to screen malignant growth utilizing dynamic reconnaissance, they look at your public service announcement like clockwork and play out a yearly DRE. What's more, they might do a recurrent biopsy and imaging in 1 to 3 years after beginning the finding.

The specialist effectively screens your side effects alone to choose if treatment is required while essentially noticing the infection.

Forceful

Specialists might treat more forceful sorts of disease with different choices, for example,
medical procedure
radiation
cryotherapy
chemical treatment
chemotherapy
stereotactic radiosurgery
immunotherapy

If your disease is exceptionally forceful and has metastasized, there's a decent opportunity it has spread to your bones. For bone metastases, the above medicines might be utilized, notwithstanding others.

Prostatectomy

A prostatectomy is a surgery that eliminates part or the entirety of your prostate organ. For instance, on the off chance that you have a prostate disease that hasn't spread beyond the prostate, your primary care physician might propose that you have an extreme prostatectomy, which eliminates the whole prostate. There are various sorts of revolutionary prostatectomies. Some are open, and that implies you'll have a bigger entry point in your lower mid-region. Others are laparoscopic, and that implies you'll have a few more modest entry points in your stomach.

Viewpoint

The viewpoint is typically great on the off chance that prostate malignant growth is analyzed early and hasn't spread from the first cancer. Early location

and treatment is basic to a positive result. Assuming you assume you have side effects of
prostate malignant growth, you ought to plan a meeting with your PCP immediately.
Notwithstanding, assuming the malignant growth advances and spreads beyond your prostate, that will influence your viewpoint.

Prostate disease anticipation

There are sure gamble factors for prostate disease, for example, age and family ancestry, that you have zero control over. In any case, there are others you can make do with.

For instance, stopping smoking could diminish your gamble of prostate malignant growth. Diet and exercise are likewise fundamental factors that can impact your gamble of prostate disease.

Diet

Certain food sources might assist with diminishing your gamble of prostate malignant growth, for example, an eating routine low in dairy and calcium. A few food varieties that could bring down your gamble of prostate disease include:

cruciferous vegetables, for example, broccoli, Brussels fledglings, and kale, fish, soy oils that contain omega-3 unsaturated fats, like olive oil

Work out

Exercise can probably assist with diminishing your gamble of creating progressed prostate malignant growth and passing on from prostate disease.

Exercise can likewise assist you with getting fitter, and it's fundamental because 2016 exploration has shown weight as a gamble factor for prostate malignant growth. With your primary care physician's endorsement, go for the gold of activity most days of the week.

Chat with your primary care physician

Prostate disease is a gamble for all men as they age, however, if it's gotten and treated early, the viewpoint is for the most part excellent. So as you age, make certain to have open discussions with your primary care physician about your gamble.

Assuming you have any side effects you think may cause prostate malignant growth, converse with your primary care physician immediately. Furthermore,

regardless of whether you have side effects, consider taking on a sound way of life to diminish your gamble.

Conclusion

Pancreatic disease is a kind of malignant growth that begins in the pancreas and can cause side effects, for example, loss of craving, unexpected weight reduction, stomach torment, blood clumps, jaundice, discouragement, light-hued or oily stools, dim or brown pee, bothersome skin, queasiness, retching, and a scope of other wellbeing concerns. Brought about by strange cells start to develop inside the pancreas and structure cancers, however it is muddled why this works out. Risk factors incorporate tobacco use, weighty liquor utilization, ongoing and inherited pancreatitis, weight, age, diabetes, race, family ancestry, contaminations, and certain hereditary varieties and changes. Early finding essentially builds the possibilities of recuperation, so it is ideal to consider a medical services proficient as soon as could be expected on the off chance that you notice any strange side effects, particularly assuming that you have any gamble factors for pancreatic malignant growth.

Pancreatic disease is a kind of malignant growth that is challenging to fix, yet therapies can assist with forestalling the spread of the disease and

straightforward side effects. Stage 3 pancreatic malignant growth is a cancer in the pancreas and conceivably close by destinations, like lymph hubs or veins. Stage 2 pancreatic malignant growth is a disease in the remaining parts of the pancreas that may have spread to a couple of neighboring lymph hubs or veins. Stage 1 pancreatic disease includes cancer that is just in the pancreas and might be treatable with medical procedures. Stage 0 pancreatic disease is the earliest phase of malignant growth, however, it may not include any side effects. Therapy for pancreatic disease includes two principal objectives: to kill malignant cells and keep the disease from spreading. Endurance rates for pancreatic disease are normally accommodated in restricted, local, and far-off stages. Racial contrasts in anticipation are driven by imbalances in therapy and long-haul racial separation, and way-of-life changes might assist with diminishing the gamble of creating pancreatic disease.

Prostate disease is the most normally analyzed malignant growth in guys around the world, with 268,490 men expected to be recently determined to have it in 2022. It is a sort of malignant growth called adenocarcinoma that fills in the tissue of an organ, like the prostate organ. It has two sorts of development: forceful, quickly developing, or slow-developing. Risk factors, for example, family ancestry or age might improve the probability of fostering the threat. Side effects of prostate disease incorporate urinary issues, sexual issues, and agony and deadness. Urinary issues incorporate the continuous need to pee a stream that is slower or more fragile than typical draining while at the same time peeing Sexual issues include erectile brokenness and blood for the semen after discharge. Torment and deadness can likewise be a side effect of prostate disease.

The main subtleties in this text are the upsides and downsides of prostate malignant growth screening. Prostate-explicit antigen (public service announcement) is a blood test that affects the number of prostate proteins in your blood, and if it is high, it might demonstrate prostate disease. A computerized rectal test (DRE) is a test that puts a greased-up, gloved finger into your rectum to feel any knocks, unbending, or expanded region of the prostate. Prostate imaging can be recognized utilizing progressed imaging, like X-ray or ultrasound. Prostate biopsy can be suggested assuming they suspect malignant growth from a test or find that they have a raised public service announcement level. The American Joint Council on Malignant Growth (AJCC) arranges framework stages of prostate disease by size or degree of cancer, lymph hub inclusion, whether the disease has spread (metastasized) to different locales or organs, public service announcement level at the hour of analysis, Gleason score, and prostate malignant growth stages range from 1 to 4. Prostate malignant growth therapy is created because of old enough, well-being status, and the phase of the disease.

The viewpoint for prostate disease is typically great on the off chance that it is analyzed early and hasn't spread from the first growth. Nonetheless, assuming the disease advances and spreads beyond the prostate, that will influence the viewpoint. To diminish the gamble of prostate malignant growth, it is critical to have standard exams with your PCP and to have open discussions with your primary care physician about your gamble. There are certain gamble factors for prostate malignant growth, for example, age and family ancestry, that can't be controlled, however, there are other gamble factors that can be made due. Exercise can assist with lessening the gamble of creating progressed prostate malignant growth and passing on from prostate disease, and regardless of whether you have side effects, consider embracing a sound way of life to diminish your gamble.

www.ingramcontent.com/pod-product-compliance
Lightning Source LLC
Chambersburg PA
CBHW070741260726
48660CB00007B/2925